ASK ANTOINETTE

A Columnist Collection of Q & A

By Antoinette Greer

ISBN: 978-1499708776
ISBN-13: 1499708777

DEDICATION

This book dedicated to my eighty-seven year old mother, who spent a great deal of her lifetime helping others and sharing what she had. While the greatest gifts are in no way monetary, they resonate in our collective passion to touch lives.

TABLE OF CONTENTS

ACKNOWLEDGMENTS

First, I would thank God for life, good health and hope in the darkest of hours; for watching over me and giving me the strength to carrying on.

I would like to acknowledge and thank those who shared their inspiration through time, talent and vision, in bringing this book to pass. For placing me in the position to deliver through availing the experiences now shared here, Toni Traylor, RN, Rachel Plotkin-Olumese, RN, BSN and Rosa Kelson of the American Cancer Society. All of whom were instrumental in assisting me with the acquisition of a support group and its programs and services.

I am ever so grateful to Jim Dooner, an individual who has constantly shown that one man can make a difference in the lives of many.

Thanks to St Mary Medical Center's staff for collaborating on events, availing space and navigational screening services to lay and vulnerable populations.

A special thanks to my Prayer Warriors, who keep me lifted in spite of life's challenges by encouraging me in knowing God has a plan for my life.

A special thanks to Dennis Holmes, M.D., for his time, talent and work in our community. He has provided guidance and direction to women battling breast cancer from start to finish.

I would further like to thank and acknowledge the Bikers Ride for Cancer riders and supporters for taking awareness to the streets to help women battling cancer meet their basic needs.

ABOUT THIS BOOK

This book is a collection of 10 questions and 10 answers previously asked of its author. It is being shared with you here and now, not as a guide or how to book, but as a columnist collection of Q and A of pivotal questions that concerned each individual who personally asked.

The advice offered in 'Ask Antoinette', as well as any advice offered by email or phone or in this book is intended for informational purposes only. Use of this book, blog, column, email or telephone to offer advice is not intended to replace or substitute for any professional, medical, legal or other professional advice. If you have specific concerns or a situation in which you need professional, psychological or medical help you should consult with a trained and licensed specialist.

Antoinette Greer is a support group facilitator and Program Coordinator at My Sister My Friend Breast Cancer Support. She offers her own personal opinions and views on a variety of subjects. She does not speak from a position of authority on any particular subject. Her opinions or views are not intended to treat or diagnose disease; nor are they intended to replace the treatment and care that you may be receiving from a licensed physician or mental health professional.

Neither is Antoinette Greer or My Sister My Friend Breast Cancer Support responsible for the outcome or results of following any advice in any given situation. Nor do they accept liability for any situation in your life's past, present or future. You and only you bear complete responsibility for your actions.

"If you talk to a man in a language he understands, that goes to his head. If you talk to him in his language, that goes to his heart."

(Nelson Mandela)

ASK ANTOINETTE

Chapter 1

WHAT CAUSED MINE?

When I decided to write this book, I wanted to start with a Frequently Asked Question (an FAQ). Not a real dynamic question but a common one for most, if not all. As most of us know cancer is not contagious but we all relish in the question "What caused mine?" Where did this cancer come from. What is normally said is "No one else in my family has it", "I exercise everyday", "and I eat right". While this good, it doesn't diminish the fact that for some reason we all received a diagnosis of cancer.

I do not believe, for me personally, that everything I ever did in life caused my breast cancer. Yes, at first in retrospect, I did take a self-inventory of my life as one would when they receive the bad news. I was sad, scared, disappointed and a bit confused. Not necessarily in that order, but I bounced off the walls every now and then at first and yes, sometimes all at once. I am a Christian by faith, but again this book is not about my take on being a Christian, so when I was diagnosed with cancer it honestly was my every thought. At some point, I came to realize what an emotional wreck I was. But this emotional wreck was normal. Somehow, all of my experiences had collided and forced me to evaluate my life and even its quality up to this point. Had I eaten poorly? Stayed up too late? Pushed too hard? Drank? Smoked? Or cursed too loud? Or was it my inherent gene pool? Was it my birth control method? Or did I hate someone or harbor ill feelings that turned into this dreadful disease? I could not answer these questions without addressing the inner conflict that I shared with nearly everyone who received this diagnosis. Medically, there are risk factors that say these things may have their root in contributory factors, whether I personally engaged in these things or not.

The Answer

I have heard various theories from professionals in the field and otherwise and although some may hold a direct correlation to me others do not. Everyone wants to help resolve the matter of facts in this question. Even though their answers may hold various truths my question was a personal one, it was about me. The truth is those of us who do not have the BRCA 1 or BRCA 2 gene mutations do not know what caused our breast cancer or why we specifically presented with the disease.

Realistically, there are variables in all of our lives that give rise to diseased states. They could range from exposure to environmental toxins, diet, lack of exercise, to a prolonged exposure to estrogen and so forth. We may all have mitigating circumstances or paradoxical proclivities that leave us wondering what exactly happened.

Rather than beat up on myself or question God or challenge that some people developed lung cancer who actually never smoked, I moved into a knowledge is power mode and faced the reality of coping with and accepting where I was now and working from there. This helped me find solution oriented fixes and presented the opportunity to correct what I could as far as my lifestyle. In this valley, I also found that people who do not know what to say should not say anything to a person who is an emotional wreck. Thus, I did not invite everyone into answering this personal question. This worked for me.

"Education is the most powerful weapon you can use to change the world."

(NELSON MANDELA)

Chapter 2

WHERE CAN I GET A GOOD THERMOGRAM?

The Question

I am a 46-year-old, African American woman who has not had a mammogram. I have a very small bump/lump/cyst, I-don't-know-what-to-call-it, above my right armpit area, above and to the right of my right breast. I am writing to you because I would really appreciate your guidance/direction/advice/experience as to where I could obtain a Thermogram? I know that some in the medical field have not fully supported Thermograms as equal to mammography technology. However, I have not gotten a mammogram because I do not want to be exposed to radiation. I know the radiation is most likely minimal, but I do know that radiation to soft tissue is carcinogenic and breasts are soft tissue.

Perhaps, the fattiest and most estrogen filled part of my body and it makes me afraid to get one. If at all possible, I would feel so relieved and at peace to obtain an accurate and reliable Thermogram. If a Thermogram is not possible, where might I get an inexpensive or no charge digital mammogram with the lowest level of radiation available and an ultrasound? Are there services or referrals you know of for someone in my situation?

I am currently unemployed and as a result, I am seeking some type of funding to offset the cost of care I deeply need. I am a USC (BA in English) and UCLA (MFA in Film) alumni. And I mention these affiliations because sometimes, those types of alliances are helpful to mention. In addition, I would offer my professional skill set to volunteer at any clinic/medical office and or support group as some sort of trade-off for discounted services. As a creative person, I am looking for a creative solution to take care of my body as a woman, seek out the care I know is available in our community and give a little something back to help someone else as well.

Thank you for taking the time to read this and offer any type of guidance, direction and or resources you may know of or have through your organization.

The Answer

I can appreciate your candid honesty. However, most of our connections are for low and no cost mammograms to women in your situation. Although, Thermograms are out there, you are correct, they do not come highly recommended by professionals in the field, particularly for women who are symptomatic e.g. have problems or symptoms as you have expressed you have. One premise is that Thermograms detect inflammation in the body based on heat and that breast tumors generate such heat. Nonetheless, my understanding was when the FDA approved such thermographic devices they were to be used in connection with mammography, as adjunct or an additional tool, not in place of. There was not sufficient evidence to support that they alone work on small or deep tumors that may go undetected. You are asking me to tell you of a "reliable" source and I cannot.

In referencing inexpensive digital mammograms, even though digital mammography is on the rise, they might not be widely used in the low and no cost arenas. Nevertheless, we can check to see if they have sliding scale fees or if there are situations and or locations where digitals might be free. You would also get a free clinical breast exam prior to the mammogram if we refer you to our contact site for these services. You would be followed annually for screening. They may even be performing digitals for free. If you are unemployed, have little or no income you should not have a problem getting a free mammogram. A trade-off would not be necessary. My advice would be to always consider whether the benefits outweigh the risks in traditional mammography. Primarily because they do and you have a problem that is now going unaddressed out of fear that the test will cause cancer. Please consider that the sooner you receive help (get screened), the more likely you are to receive a good resolve and treatment if you have cancer; the sooner the better your outcome.

I hope this helps.

The Resolve
The Writer did obtain a mammogram.

Antoinette's Response

I am happy to hear you have made a good and informed decision. As a 10 ½ year breast cancer survivor (at the time), the pivotal gain for me was an ultimate impact on my life's expectancy. I chose life and have since then learned that the ministry I am gifted with is not just for me. I wish you all the best.

Author's Notes

We are empowered to impart knowledge to each other and seek out solutions to common problems if and when we speak on them. Suffering in silence is not an option. Become a part of the solution, stay in touch with your breast and resolve problems early. Perform monthly Breast Self Exams and get a visual.

WHAT IS THERMOGRAPHY (THERMAL IMAGING)?

According to the American Cancer Society "Thermography" is:

"A way to measure and map the heat on the surface of the breast using a special heat-sensing camera. It's based on the idea that the temperature rises in areas with increased blood flow and metabolism, which could be a sign of a tumor."

Thermography has been around for many years, but studies have shown that it's not an effective screening tool for finding breast cancer early. Although it has been promoted as helping detect breast cancer early, a 2012 research review found that thermography was able to detect only a quarter of the breast cancers found by mammography. In other words, it failed to detect 3 out of 4 cancers that were known to be present in the breast. Digital infrared thermal imaging (DITI), which some people believe is a newer and better type of thermography, has the same failure rate. This is why thermography should not be used as a substitute for mammograms.[ii]

WHAT ARE THE SYMPTOMS?

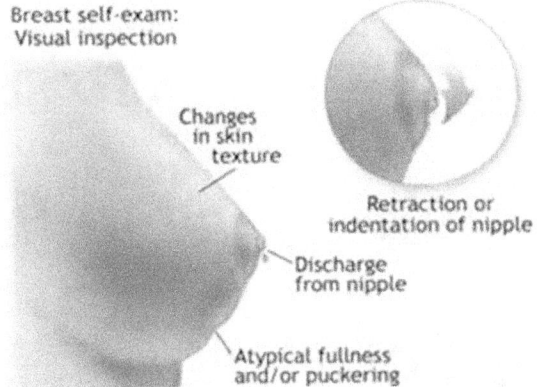

Breast self-exam:
Visual inspection

Changes in skin texture

Retraction or indentation of nipple

Discharge from nipple

Atypical fullness and/or puckering

The symptoms of breast cancer include:

1. A lump or thickening in or near the breast or in the underarm that persists through the menstrual cycle.
2. A mass or lump, which may feel as small as a pea.
3. A change in the size, shape or contour of the breast.
4. A blood-stained or clear fluid discharge from the nipple.
5. A change in the feel or appearance of the skin on the breast or nipple (dimpled, puckered, scaly or inflamed).
6. Redness of the skin on the breast or nipple.
7. A change in shape or position of the nipple.
8. An area that is distinctly different from any other area on either breast.
9. A marble-like hardened area under the skin.[iii]

Any one of these nine symptoms shows cause for you to visit a doctor, get screened and obtain a professional opinion.

"The best place to find a helping hand is at the end of your arm."

SWEDISH PROVERB

CHAPTER 3

BORING BRAS, NOT VICKY'S SECRET

I was wondering what I could do? I shop for my prosthesis at the retailers that were listed in the information from my doctor. The prosthetic bras I find are in three basic colors black, beige and white. These are boring, not sexy colors; I was a Vicky Secret (Victoria Secret) shopper and fan prior to my cancer. Most of the bras I like have under wires and I've heard rumors they can cause breast cancer. I tried putting my prosthesis in regular bras but don't feel secure. What options do I have?

Bored but Sexy, Cerritos, CA

The Answer

I would imagine you would feel less secure as regular (non-prosthetic) bras don't have pockets for the prosthesis. They can sometimes reveal it or by it being less secure, it might shift as you move and go about your day. There is some controversy over underwire bras and breast cancer for various reasons. Rather than elaborate on those reasons and the studies surrounding them, I would say for women who choose to wear underwire type bras, relieve your stress and remove the wire. Remove the underwire through making a small slit under the corner of the bra and sliding the metal (wire) out.

Bras that fit properly give women a sense of security (in appearance, posture and proper circulation), that I believe you're looking for and they tend to support the shoulders and back. They work for me.

Now, back to your concern of colorful and sexy mastectomy bras. Yes, most retailers do only have three possibly four colors. See if one of your options on the list from your doctor's is Nordstrom. It was on the list of retailers from my doctor. I shop at Nordstrom and with their Prosthesis Program; they will pocket any bras you choose from the entire selection of bras in their lingerie department. They also have bra fitters and fitting events for women who wear prosthesis. Visit their website and check out their prosthesis program at: //shop.nordstrom.com/c/prosthesis-program.

Stay Sexy and Exciting!
Antoinette

"Nowadays people know the price of everything and the value of nothing"

(OSCAR WILDE)

Chapter 4

ARE SUPPORT GROUPS SELF-HELP?

Yes, support groups are a form of self-help when they are peer led. The peer is usually not a professional counselor or therapist in traditional peer led support group settings but normally shares the same or a similar burdensome condition or characteristics of its members. These group types present various opportunities to learn from each participant's experiences, support networks and are storehouses of resourceful information. Wikipedia defines a self-help support group as:

> *"Fully organized and managed by its members, who are commonly volunteers and have personal experience in the subject of the group's focus. These groups may also be referred to as fellowships, peer support groups, lay organizations, mutual help groups or mutual aid self-help groups."*

On the other hand, it defines professionally operated support groups as:

> *"Facilitated by professionals who most often do not share the problem of the members, [1] such as social workers, psychologists or members of the clergy. The facilitator controls discussions and provides other managerial service. Such professionally operated groups are often found in institutional settings, including hospitals,*

drug-treatment centers and correctional facilities. These types of support group may run for a specified period of time and an attendance fee is sometimes charged."

Most women battling breast cancer can appreciate both a peer setting and or a professional support group in terms of seeking out information and emotional release amongst attendees. Cultural competence is generally sought out as an important factor in choosing a lasting support group setting, as well as a specific cancer type. For instance, groups that are broad in supporting all cancer types may not yield as many breast cancer survivor women with female cancer types as regular attendees to its meetings alongside men treating for other cancers.

Question (Part 2)

I ASKED BECAUSE A FAMILY MEMBER HAS BREAST CANCER; HOW CAN I GET HER INVOLVED IN A SUPPORT GROUP?

You be supportive to her in the meantime and take the time to find out if she wants a support group setting for herself. Or get clear on if she wants outside support at all. You can want it for her. Yet, she needs to want it for herself. Most people have some idea of what to expect to receive from a group or how they envision support groups overall. Or maybe she has trouble coping with or grasping her troubled state in the present time. Her views could be skewed by a number of things and mixed emotions. Be it good or bad, they could be based on her individualized perception of what she thinks about these groups. Or maybe just the concept of what she thinks she needs in the moment. Mainly, if she has never participated or been exposed to what happens in support group settings. My elderly mother has an interesting way of putting things when they happen suddenly or when we (her children) need a quick response or decision from her. She simply says, "You're taking me too fast." My mom is eighty seven years old and we do get it. It takes time to decide.

When I took the step to start attending support groups upon my diagnosis, I could appreciate my need to find people who knew how I felt. I didn't have any other expectations; rather, I felt the need to see some people who looked like me who were surviving the disease. In my case, it was totally my decision. I think we all have some idea of how sick people should feel, but we could be wrong.

I have heard many women who attended our groups say they thought it was going to be depressing and that indirectly, there would be some preoccupation with death from the disease. This was a perception and not the reality once they attended a support group. Find out if she wants outside support at all. You are there with her, be supportive, but she has to want other support. If you need support and are caring for her directly join a support group for caregivers.

Having said all this, support groups are excellent sources of information and support. They may also yield advocacy and various other benefits long term. Nonetheless, they are not the only form of support. Often, church goers find support through their clergy members, social groups, friends and family. This may be individualized and not in a group setting. It is still support.

I often receive calls from someone whose relative has breast cancer and they want to know how to get the person who has cancer to come to a support group meeting. Suggest it and see what kind of response you get. Most support groups for cancer will generally be offered by hospitals and clinics where one receives their treatment, even if they are not the vehicle directly providing the service.

Aside from cancer groups, groups that deal with Alcohol and Drug Counseling will more than likely tell the family member to have the person dealing with the problem/disease to contact them directly. This is to ensure they want this type of support for themselves. After all, they will be the one attending and following through with their treatment plans and services. It doesn't make sense that anyone would or should force their participation.

"For I know the plans I have for you," declares the LORD, *"plans to prosper you and not to harm you, plans to give you hope and a future."*

Jeremiah 29:11 (NIV)

Chapter 5

SHOULD PEOPLE WHO HAVE FAITH IN GOD GO TO THE DOCTOR WHEN THEY GET SICK?

Yes, they should. The question posed here is essentially, "Should my healing be divine?" A friend once shared what happened with first lady, Dr. Betty Price and Dr. Betty's cancer. In fact, she gave me Dr. Betty's book titled, *Through the Fire & Through the Water; My Triumph Over Cancer"*. Dr. Betty was diagnosed with lymphoma. My summation of her story is she thought God would heal her miraculously, without the aid of doctors or medicine. What Dr. Betty eventually saw was that God was going to operate through people, not the way she anticipated He would initially. Until she accepted this fact, she would not find relief or remedy in anything she tried. I still say it was by divine revelation that she ultimately grasps this. She went to the doctor and was treated. Praise God for her revelation. Thank God she got the message in time. Did prayer and intercessory help? Does God answer prayer? The answer is yes to both of these questions.

Upon my diagnosis, my sister Cheryl believed I needed to visit churches for an instant healing (the Laying on of Hands). She had me go with her to about two, until I realized what she was doing. I knew in her heart she meant well. She was scared for me. My sister Alfreda had recently died after being diagnosed with COPD (Chronic Obstructive Pulmonary Disease). My family had all watched at her hospital bedside as she unconsciously wasted away, in the last thirty days of her life, one year prior to my diagnosis. Alfreda was forty-four years of age when she died.

I believe my relationship with God is personal and my prayers were fervent. I explained to my sister that I already have God and He is on my side. God operates as He chooses. If He chooses, when He chooses, where He chooses and who He chooses to operate through, if He chooses anyone at all. I believed in my case, He would operate through people, so I did believe I needed doctors and surgery. I had not prayed my mass/tumor away. I had already made that attempt. I exercised my faith. I had prayed vigorously while I was awaiting my test results, but nonetheless, the results were what they were. And I do believe God heard me. Chemotherapy was not at the top of the list of my desires either. Can God heal miraculously? Yes, He can, when and if He chooses. The bible specifically says when we are sick we should go to the elders of the church and asked for prayer. I followed this instruction also.

There are three major points I would like to make. One is that as humans on both a spiritual and physical journey, we have a tendency to wrestle with justice and judgment, all within the scope of a limited understanding. Specifically, when we are disappointed, when we are in pain or when we receive instructions or answers that don't feel good. Our first rationalization efforts are rooted in why this happened in the first place. The scripture says that not all sickness is due to sin, but for God to get the glory (John 9), which further supports that we might not know the reason why. We find further passages that support God's power as the life force and the ultimate authority as in the book of Job; wherein sickness, pain and loss paint a very different and unique picture. The paradox is that Job is sick not because he was bad, but because he was good. The scripture does not tell us that he ever personally knew why he was sick or whether he went to the doctor to recover. In either case, we know that God was with him. Randy Alcorn, Best Selling Author of *Heaven*, touched on this in his book titled, *If God is Good Why Do We Hurt?* When he offers:

"Often, as I've contemplated potentially faith-jarring situations and sought His truth, God has wiped away my own tears, while my journey hasn't unearthed easy answers; I'm astonished at how much insight scripture offers. And after much wrestling with the issues, instead of being disheartened, I have hope".

Secondly, does God have a need for doctors? When we go to scripture, we find that Luke was a physician. Luke is poised as an Apostle, with Paul. Luke is credited with being the author of both Acts and the gospel of Luke. Therein, we also find Jesus healing through miracles and sometimes with methods included. He used mud on the blind man's eyes (John 9). Do we know why He used it? No, we don't.

Lastly, God also operates in both the natural and the spiritual realm. He is not limited to space or time. He has provided tools and technology whereby its use is primarily good.

At some point, I had begun to pray for guidance, support and the right vessels attending to my condition. I would hate to think that I got to heaven early because God didn't show up looking like I thought He should. And for Him to tell me "I sent you a team of doctors and you refused their help". I was at peace with God's answers and my choices. To this day, I believe my healing was and is, divine. I now walk in divine healing. My sister now calls it a faith walk. It was not a cake walk but a faith walk, I would tend to agree.

I was diagnosed with a 4.5 centimeter, high grade tumor as a Stage III over twelve years ago. The treatment involved four methods and the entire process took one year. Therein lies the miracle.

"Love isn't something you find. Love is something that finds you."

(Loretta Young)

Chapter 6

SHOULD I TELL A POTENTIAL MATE ABOUT MY CANCER EXPERIENCE?

My answer is "I would". Why? Because good, healthy relationships are built on honesty, trust and good communication.

Some women take the position that a history of breast cancer will scare men away. Their biggest fear is rejection. Yes, it could scare him away, but again, that is a matter of what he perceives your health history to mean. I personally would ask myself if it were better to let him know prior to developing any emotional attachments. This way, there is no real risk of being heartbroken if it posed a problem later, if and when he found out. I think some of us may have esteem issues. Often times, emotional baggage is rooted in how we feel about ourselves and what we think no one else would want or what people actually tell us they don't want. In my experience, most men would want to know just as we would want to know about their health history. Any man who I had personally told only asked, "Are you alright now?" which is a good relative question to right now, in the present. Not so much what happened to me, but where I am now.

I also say to know your comfort zone. When to tell may be a bigger challenge for some. Hiding generally does not help matters. Hiding things is the same as omission. Omission in relationships is generally categorized with lies or things that are not so good. When we find out things that have been omitted, we tend to have trust issues with the person who left it out. Keeping secrets is hard. It's like sitting on the lid of Pandora's Box and it takes work as one would have to stay guarded so the secret doesn't get out. Who has that kind of time or energy? And in doing so, we entertain a series of "what if" questions. Again, fear is typically at the core of hiding. Usually, when we start explaining what we left out, we start our sentences with, "I didn't tell you because I was afraid that......"

On another note, the situation often arises where women have scares with a fear that cancer might have returned. In these situations, most of us would vie for the support of our counterparts and not want instances where we could not discuss this with those around us, specifically our mates. In loving and caring relationships, we should be able to talk about anything, especially our problems. One would attempt to seek comfort there first, but how could we if we never told? On the other hand, if it scares the man away, for me, it would be good to know early. Therefore, I have not invested a lot of time in someone who is not the right person or in things that don't work. If it's a deal breaker, so to speak, for him, I would love to know early.

After I answered this question, I found an article on the same topic online. It was in a blog forum and the man who was asked the question about when "a woman should tell", expressed feeling awkward about being asked because he was a man. Secondly, he wrote that he felt there was no right time to tell and that regardless of when you told, it would be good to "steel" yourself from possible rejection. For me, rejection would be defined as redirection.

Remember, the question is not about telling everyone, but about a potential mate. Everyone we date might not fit in this category right off the bat. How many dates would make him a potential mate? At some point in a relationship, one will engage in intimacy with their mate. Most of us have surgery scars from treating for the disease, which may more than likely become a topic of conversation. Even if you had reconstruction, unless you sleep in your bra, most breasts are not without some sort of scaring or difference from the other breast. If you had a mastectomy, without reconstruction, there will be no breast there at all. Again, of course, unless you kept your bra on, he would notice.

On the flip side of the coin, there are stories we hear whereby the man left after learning about the diagnoses at the inception of their mate being diagnosed with breast cancer. Again, even though this is obviously a dreadful situation, we have to ask ourselves if he was the right mate in the first place. Would the person for me not be there for me in sickness and in health? This would not be a good time to find out he's not the right one.

A friend once asked me how I would personally tell a man because she and I are both single African American women and survivors. She said she doesn't tell. I am a very private person, or at least I would like to believe I am. My response was, "It's what I do, how could I not tell?" Adding, "I run a support group for women with the disease." If I didn't tell, what could I tell him later if he found out? "Oh, you never asked." Why would we need to have this conversation at all? The truth is, I wouldn't care what he thinks, in a sense that if we just met and it scares you off. You are not for me. I would want to know now. What works for me may not work for you. I am not my breasts and would need someone to love me, like it or not. Ultimately, I would like to think that, at the end of the day, what we are all seeking is love, marriage at some point, lifelong companionship and not just a Facebook Fan. With love comes accepting real people for who they really are. For me, companionship requires compatibility. The definition of the word means "well-matched" or "well suited", so be it a quality relationship. I love who I am and most things about me. My truths are my truths. If the person is well-suited for me, it won't be a deal breaker. I have not heard any real horror stories from my friend; praise God, she is still in good health. She is single, dating and in hiding. Apparently, her perspective works for her. If you need help with any decision-making or working through interpersonal relationship conflicts and the myriad of mixed emotions that go along with them, talk to someone (seek professional counseling).

"What lies behind us and what lies before us are tiny matters compared to what lies within us."

(Ralph Waldo Emerson)

Chapter 7

IS RECONSTRUCTION RIGHT FOR ME?

A positive body image is very important to the mental and emotional health of those affected by breast cancer, generally speaking, who we are and how we are is often rooted in how we feel about ourselves inwardly. Remnants of this rises to the surface by way of our personality traits and in our dealings with others within our social settings. The comingling of these factors influences how we develop socially and all of which may have an effect on our self-esteem. Let's face it, today, in America, for some, breasts are a symbol of femininity, sexiness, motherhood and so forth. In addition, breasts are big business, especially here in Southern California. Surrounded by sun and beach cities, California is known for its glitz, glamour and Hollywood. Hollywood is noteworthy for being cosmetically correct. Those with healthy breasts get them augmented for a significant price. As you consider getting your breast reconstruction some pressing questions and feelings may arise. To help answer these questions, do seek to include those with experience in these areas in your decision making.

In my opinion, you should ask your doctors what options are available to you specifically. This is not so much about costs or health plans and benefits. For most, treating patients and survivors of breast cancer there is no charge. These services are free. They are deemed a part of their course of treatment. Availability lies in various factors specific to the individual. Options vary by patient size, breast shape and breast size, whether or not radiotherapy is needed, previous abdominal surgeries, co-morbidities and other risk factors (e.g., smoking). For instance, if one has a history of heart attacks they would more than likely not be a good candidate for the Tram Flap (a breast formed from their stomach fat and or muscle, or the Back Flap (a breast formed from their back muscle). While there are other flap types, most if not all of these surgery types are very extensive and require hours of being under anesthesia during the process. There is notable strength loss from procedures that involve taking muscles. Thus, the possibility of obtaining one where the muscle is spared is called "free". Sparing the muscle may reduce some of the risks of abdominal complications for those taken from the stomach area. There is also what is known as a Diep Flap (Deep Inferior Epigastric Perforator Flap). This procedure is fairly new and described as replacing these other flaps, but because of longer operative time, limited reimbursement, the need for ICU care and overall expense, many plastic surgeons and hospitals are backing off of doing DIEPs. So, patients should shop around, especially if they do not have "good" insurance.

Sources of information can be found online that can help you develop questions to ask your doctor:

http://www.mayoclinic.org/tests-procedures/breast-reconstruction/ basics/what-you-can-expect/prc-20020499http://prma-enhance.com/ breast-reconstruction/tram-flap

Ask your doctor to explain the differences in such surgeries and both the short and long term side-effects of each and what they mean to you specifically. Ask about the recovery period, risks and possible additional surgeries required to complete the job before you start. There will typically be more than one surgical procedure required to complete reconstruction. How many depends on the type selected and other factors. Skin grafts might be required from other areas of the body. A tattoo for the areola is typically required, but not needed in a nipple sparing mastectomy.

Whether or not you have had radiation therapy in the chest area may also be a factor in the quality or the appearance at the outcome.

Radiation tends to create scar tissue and toughens the skin. The skin may not stretch adequately enough over a silicone or saline implant. Thus, it may appear pulled or require grafting skin from other places. In the setting of post-mastectomy radiotherapy most plastic surgeons prefer tissue flap reconstructions.

What may matter in all cases is what you would deem feasible or worth it when examining overall satisfaction at the final outcome. Embracing your *"New Normal"*, is first to understand exactly what will be "normal" for you.

Do some research and share whatever your anticipation is with your surgeon to get a realistic view of what you can expect at the outcome. Many women have heightened levels of expectations and some are happy whereas others may be largely disappointed. Ask to see pictures of before and after of others who have had similar surgery types. Ask if there are any videos in the office that you may view or for access to other women who have had similar surgeries to gain their satisfaction after their process was complete. Join a support group or visit one, to obtain answers from women who have had different kinds of reconstructive breast surgeries. However, always be mindful that no two people are exactly the same and satisfaction levels will vary accordingly.

Some women opt to use their own body fat and or muscle whereas others choose implants. Some choose not to get breast reconstruction at all and simply wear a prosthetic breast. It is whatever works for the individual. I support whatever you choose. Again, ask these questions. You are your best advocate. Make an informed decision.

"We can easily forgive a child who is afraid of the dark; the real tragedy of life is when men are afraid of the light."

(PLATO)

Chapter 8

I HAVE A FEAR OF CANCER RETURNING WHAT SHOULD I DO?

Fear of recurrence is normal for most cancer survivors[v]. Primarily, when all treatment has concluded, some patients feel that they must continue to see doctors outside of the suggested norm of treatment protocols and follow-up care recommendations, for some reassurance that cancer is in fact gone. This safety net is mostly the psychological impact of being diagnosed and treated for the disease. Initially, one has a team of doctors, which speaks to the seriousness of one's condition.

For instance, when the doctor tells you, 'I will see you in one year', some women become very disturbed and want to know if this is right. The feeling is 'I need you to see me to make sure I'm okay and that the cancer is really gone.' The real assurance is if you feel you have a problem or become symptomatic, you are free to schedule an appointment to visit this doctor any time and not await your annual appointment. As a support group leader and a cancer survivor I have heard and had many relative experiences. I followed all the treatment protocols and follow-up appointments, but when I felt there was something wrong or not quite right, I scheduled an appointment and gained the attention of my doctor and got the benefit of a professional opinion. I, too, have had scares. At first, I lived in the safe zone. There was nothing wrong with living there when I needed to. I never ignored anything I felt was a problem and neither should you. In fact, the American Cancer Society has an excellent article on their website about mixed emotions after completing treatment for cancer types that can recur. It's titled, *"Living With Uncertainty: The Fear of Cancer Recurrence"* at http://www.cancer.org.

After my Chemo and Radiation treatments were done, I followed with Tamoxifen for five years. I had estrogen receptor positive cancer. Not all women diagnosed with breast cancer have estrogen receptor positive tumors. Therefore, every woman is not prescribed Tamoxifen. I was pre-menopausal when I diagnosed, as I was only forty years old. I was actually glad when my treatment was over, but I did have scares; being a part of a support group helped me know that I was not alone. When I got sick with anything other than a cold or flu, my first thought was they (doctors) are always going to look for cancer. After all, I do have a cancer history now, but often times I was wrong.

I had to, at some point, realize I needed to cope with this very real fear when something did come up. Even when undergoing tests to find out if the cancer had recurred. It was during this process and after, I learned what could help me avoid recurrence by researching breast cancer survivors and recurrent risk reduction methods. First, I found that people with cancer overall lived longer when they had support of some sort. Although I wasn't seeking to know this, it was good to know. I then learned that an exercise as simple as walking would help reduce recurrent risks. I, thereafter, gave my attention to what I already knew about optimal health and balance. I knew that a nutrient dense diet would also reduce risks and would aid in warding off cancer's return. I figured this was simple and the least I could do. I would replace worry with a kind of productivity and reward. My suggestion to you is to cut out or at least cut down on behaviors that contribute to diseased states by making positive lifestyle changes. Avoid or minimize your intake of processed foods, fried foods and items with high calorie content but no nutritional value like soft drinks. Eat lots of leafy green vegetables, fresh fruits, whole grains, legumes and lean meats. Don't overcook vegetables, but steam them or eat them raw. Find healthier alternatives to ingredients in the foods you normally eat. An excellent place to find recipe alternatives is Kitchen Divas, a program offered through Black Women for Wellness, an organization based in Los Angeles, California. Also, get into the habit of exercising. Walk for at least 30 minutes a day or take a dance class. Make it something you enjoy. Pair up with friends or neighbors and develop a routine. Exercise helps in more ways than one and quality sleep rejuvenates the body. In all cases, an ounce of prevention is worth a pound of cure.

My findings as a support group facilitator are that when most women recurred or entertained its scares within our support group setting, they did not want anyone else to know. Even though they didn't always yet know the outcome of such test results, they would share with me only. One claim was they did not want to burden their families. Although I respect everyone's wishes, my question is, "How can you be supported if no one knows?" It is not to say you need to tell everyone. How can you help us help you? The biggest hurdle to climb is that others might be negative regarding your perceived outcome. Therefore, it does pay to be conservative and very selective concerning who you tell what to. When and if cancer returns the outcome does not have to be a negative one. Nonetheless, it is true that the perception of others might be negative. Always be mindful that you are responsible for your own perceptions, thoughts and ideas and that you must guard them. If you need professional help with coping, seek help and get help. Whatever you decide, do not allow fear to immobilize you.

I knew a woman whose breast cancer returned five years after her initial treatment concluded. She had bone metastasis. She lived another twenty years, a very positive person during treatment intervals and otherwise, with a good quality of life. Be mindful that everyone is different and every situation is unique. Everyone's cancer will not return; neither do we need to live in fear. Stress and worry only complicate things. Life will get back to some normalcy. Take care of yourself by doing what you can to reduce your risks; get follow-up care as prescribed and medical attention when needed and stay positive.

"Your talent is God's gift to you. What you do with it is your gift back to God".

(Leo Buscaglia)

Chapter 9

SHOULD I TAKE HERBAL SUPPLEMENTS DURING TREATMENT?

My answer to this question would vary depending on several factors. I think one would first need to define and differentiate between "complementary" and "alternative" medicines and conventional medicines. On one hand, complementary means to "complement" something and is usually done in addition to or "paired with". The other term, in contrast means "instead of" (alternative) in place of or "unconventional". I often find people tend to confuse these terms and use them interchangeably. Conventional would mean mainstream medicine.

You would also need to make a distinction in the choice and or purpose of what they are attempting to achieve. If the intent is to replace treatment all together with alternative type supplements and therapies, be clear on two facts. One is just because it is an herb or natural supplement does not mean it does not come with adverse side effects from its use. Two is that medicines are normally derived from plant sources, but come with controlled, prescribed use/dosages based on scientific data. Although the other (herbal supplements) may have limitations in use, such limitations are unknown because of the lack of scientific data. Conventional medicines are put to various trials, studies, i.e., research, whereas most herbs are not. There are also some controversial herbs concerning to their influence on estrogen in female cancers.

Thus, my answer in the complementary sense would be based upon the type of cancer treatment you are undergoing at the time. If you are undergoing adjuvant therapies such as chemotherapy or taking conventional medicines, you should beware of additional factors. Keep in mind the very intent of these therapies is to kill cancer cells, shrink tumors, inhibit estrogen and so forth. Chemotherapy works best on actively growing cells. Things that slow cancer's growth might inhibit chemotherapy, leaving you with the side effects, but little benefit from treatment. If the supplement would interfere with the intent of a cancer treating therapy, it would be best to wait until after your chemo is over. Otherwise, what good would treatment serve? Always keep your doctors informed and gain clearance through them that the supplement is okay to take during treatment by them.

Although, there have been a variety of research studies on herbs and cancer, there are very few, if any, that I know of that have conclusive findings. This is probably why the FDA (Food & Drug Administration) warns and restricts companies when making therapeutic claims on their packaging, websites and in their marketing materials that they cure disease in all cases, when and if there is no scientific data to support and/or demonstrate safe and effective use. Though some consumers may not trust pharmaceutical companies, these companies do invest large amounts of money in testing and research of their drugs. They also have to comply with the FDA in submitting evidence based findings through scientific data as mentioned above[vi].

Herbal remedies such as Chinese Herbal Medicines have been around for ages and have their roots in traditional Chinese Culture. The American Cancer Society has an online article (@http://www.cancer.org/treatment/treatmentsandsideeffects/com plementaryandalternativemedicine/herbsvitaminsandminerals/chines e-herbal-medicine) on the subject to include an overview, the history, what's involved, promotion, the evidence and complications. I believe that some herbal supplements may have some benefit.

However, those benefits would be difficult to measure in uncontrolled environments. I haven't personally witnessed any of them cure cancer.

Confusing the Holistic Approach

The holistic approach is an acclimated lifestyle change and not merely the taking of herbal supplements or the use of home remedies or antidotes. This approach includes involving the physical, mental, emotional and spiritual state of an individual in an effort to create or restore a natural balance. It is considered a mind-body approach. Nonetheless, the quality of an individual's experiences bears a direct correlation with achieving such balance. It would have to include the socioeconomic status of the individual bartering what the individual has at their disposal in terms of resources. The Cultural Dictionary defines 'Socioeconomic Status' as:

"An individual's or group's position within a hierarchical social structure. Socioeconomic status depends on a combination of variables, including occupation, education, income, wealth and place of residence. Sociologists often use socioeconomic status as a means of predicting behavior."[vii]

The American Psychological Association defines Socioeconomic Status (SES) as:

"Socioeconomic status is commonly conceptualized as the social standing or class of an individual or group. It is often measured as a combination of education, income and occupation. Examinations of socioeconomic status often reveal inequities in access to resources, plus issues related to privilege, power and control."[viii]

Take my mother, for example. My mother is eighty-seven years old and from the Deep South Isola, Mississippi. My mother was born in 1927 and came to California in 1957. For Blacks in the South, they didn't have much by the way of doctors or medicines. Back then, doctors, if you could get one, actually made house calls. In fact, my mother said that when the doctor came, he only had two bottles of medicine, one red and one white. My mother gave birth to twelve children, mostly through midwives. My mother knew of her father, but was raised by her aunt because her mother died when she was six years old. At times, growing up she lived on plantations, where whites housed their workers after the war. Often times, other sections of these houses were occupied by other black families who were strangers simply seeking the same work and refuge.

Here is an illustration of a home remedy and limited resources. My mother shared with me that when she was a little girl, she had an incident once where she stepped on a rusty nail. Her aunt tore a clean white cloth in half, took a piece of salt pork and with the cloth, tied the salt pork to the wound to draw the poison out, because they had no Tetanus shots. Tetanus, also known as Lockjaw is a disease that affects the nervous system and leads to spasms.[ix] Today, we could and would simply go to a doctor and get the shot. The shot lasts for ten years.

Although, they were all adamant church goers back then, their essential diets were high in sodium, animal fat and lard was used for cooking; exercise was namely field or day (domestic) work and stress levels remained heightened based on societal deficiencies of this era. Today, the average cost of a holistic retreat for cancer or other degenerative disease treatment alternatives ranges from $2,900 to $4,500 per week. Most combine a conventional medical assessment and treatment with alternative medical diagnostics and what is categorized as healing therapies.

Today, we can make healthier lifestyle choices while integrating some changes in mind-body balance within the scope of our individual resources.

Personally, it was my experience that everyone seemed to have the magic bullet when I was diagnosed with breast cancer, advising me on what I should be doing or taking to enhance my body's ability to fight the disease. Although they meant well, I had to make an informed decision for myself what my treatment course would entail. I think I heard a million times "drink this" or "eat that", "for your immune system" or "for energy". "Go on a raw food diet and juice everything". What I actually learned, by reading and from my doctors during treatment, was that with a low white blood count and a compromised immune as a result of treatment, I should stay away from certain raw foods because of their bacteria content and my inability to fight it off during chemotherapy.[x] This would help me avoid infection. So, what appeared to be good advice from Aunt Sarah and Uncle Rob was actually bad, considering my immediate state. I stopped dining out all together at the time. Under normal circumstances, I would have possessed the ability to fight bad bacteria. Therefore, tolerable cooked food became my friend for the time being. Five days after each chemo session, I had a low white blood count and needed a shot of Neupogen to prompt my bone marrow to create white blood cells. These cells would help me fight infection. This was continuously measured by routine blood work. I elected to give myself shots at home.

One day, while in treatment for the disease, I was sitting in the waiting room at my doctor's office. I encountered an elderly Caucasian woman who had cervical cancer. Her cancer was stage IV. We engaged in conversation and maybe twenty minutes into it, she asked me what else I was doing for my cancer. I was somewhat bewildered by the question and couldn't respond immediately. I wrestled with the meaning of the question at first. She went on to explain that she had spent $5,000 on some pills that were supposed to cure her. She said, "I am feeling better, too." I asked her if she told her doctor about these pills and she answered, "No, I'm not going to." She shared that she did not know what was in the pills. When she asked me again, "What else are you doing (besides treatment)?" While the question for me was still somewhat perplexing, all that came to mind was to answer "Other than getting treatment, I'm praying," adding, "That's what I'm doing; I'm praying". Although I sympathized with the woman, I seriously couldn't fathom paying $5,000 for something and not even know what it was or be ingesting it, be it a placebo or not. I would at least need to know the ingredients, even if I had $5,000. This woman never asked for my advice. I merely asked her, "What if what you are taking interferes with your treatment?" She didn't really answer the question and it was as though her intent was to advise me to get some of these pills. I just listened. Me, I had lost my income during treatment. Meeting basic needs became a top priority when that happened and I wasn't interested in purchasing those pills or adding any other supplements to my treatment. The receptionist called my name as the doctor was ready to see me and thus concluded our conversation.

My advice is whatever you choose to add to treatment or replace it with, know what's in it, what's involved and the possible side effects. Whether it is an overload of vitamins, herbal supplements, therapies, enemas, concoctions, drinks, shakes, pills or other home remedies, it is critical that you know what you are ingesting. Do some research and share it with your doctors. Again, it is by personal choice that one does whatever he or she elects to do in treating their disease. Do make informed decisions. It is not to say your choice would not be supported but not knowing could be counterproductive.

The Conspiracy Theory

I am not one who believes there is a conspiracy theory, that the doctors have a cure for the disease, but won't share it because of pharmaceutical companies or monetary gain. I believe cancer to be a complex disease with many forms and self-sustaining factors. I also believe that medicine has come a long way in seeking to cure or to arrest the disease. Although I do understand the desperation to be cured, the offering of that from love ones and that there is and always will be others who prey on the very fact that we all desire a cure so greatly.

Author's Notes

Although raising twelve children in the inner city comes with its own situational stressors, overall, my parents fared well after transitioning to California in the late '50's. With solid work ethics, my father achieved employment with Hughes Aircraft and later, General Motors. They purchased two homes. My mother, as a homemaker, grew her own garden, cultivated the soil for vegetables and fruits; raised chickens, rabbits and pigeons. Although, we only ate the vegetables and fruits, we grew up having had well-rounded experiences. My mother later worked outside the home and retired from King-Drew Hospital. My mother was also diagnosed with breast cancer when I was sixteen years old. One of my younger brothers had renal failure by the age of eighteen, secondary due to high blood pressure. The reality is our socioeconomic status and environmental factors influenced our life's quality. We, therefore, must work at incorporating healthier lifestyle changes to achieve balance and wholeness for optimal health.

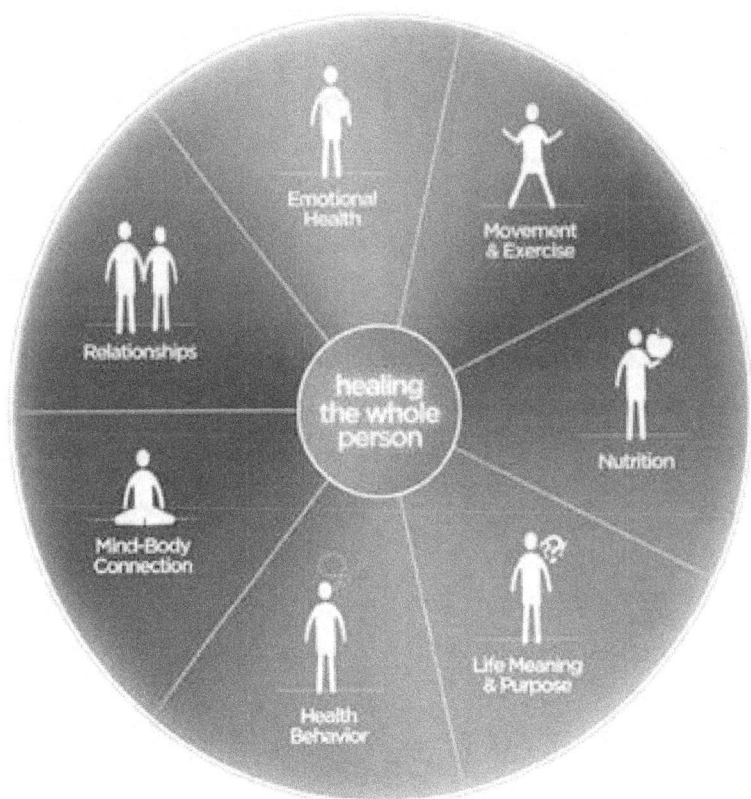

I was an avid herbal supplement taker at various intervals throughout my life. I chose to take certain supplements only after researching their benefits and learning how to use them. I educated myself, through obtaining various books on their use, benefits and side effects. I also found that most nutritional based study results and findings came from the real food sources and not supplements. I decided, however, that while treating for cancer, I would refrain from taking these supplements. I took a multiple vitamin and opted to make different and more lifestyle changes when I struggled with the fear of recurrence. During treatment, like most cancer patients in chemotherapy, I had eating problems which included nausea and constipation side effects at times. Some women get mouth sores and diarrhea as side effects during treatment. My sense of smell and taste were off, which adversely affected my appetite and stomach. Like most treating cancer patients I experienced lots of fatigue and a loss of appetite. I did drink mint and green herbal teas at times, when challenged with stomach problems.

Prior to being diagnosed with breast cancer, I exercised regularly, ate mostly fish, chicken and turkey, no red meat. I did not eat fried foods or processed junk foods like chips or drink sodas. I consumed very little sweets and my diet included a variety of vegetables and fruits. I consumed most starches in their pure forms and brown rice. I juiced regularly and typically ate two meals per day. I'm five feet 10 inches tall and maintained a weight on average of one hundred and fifty pounds. I do know that not everyone starts here, but we all have to start somewhere to cultivate change for better outcomes.

"Love recognizes no barriers. It jumps hurdles, leaps fences, penetrates walls to arrive at its destination full of hope."

(Maya Angelou)

Chapter 10

WHAT DOES METASTASIS MEAN?

Metastasis means 'to spread" cancer cells from one organ of the body to another. Metastatic Breast Cancer is defined as breast cancer that has spread to one or more parts of the body. Often times, it is referred to in short as *"mets"*. This does not normally include when such cancer is found in the armpit lymph nodes near the cancer. The lymph nodes are identified as such because they are a component of the lymphatic system, a system known for helping the body clear waste and fight infectious diseases. The lymphatic system runs throughout the body. This system acts as a significant part in the health of the body's immune system.[xi] Medical findings suggest that it is through this system and/or the circulatory system that cancer spreads to other parts of the body. This is why the first surgery usually involves removal of the lymph nodes in the armpit area closest to the breast where the cancer was found to detect signs of cancer's spread.

For the purpose of clarity, I often hear women say, when cancer spreads to another area of the body, that it took on the identity of that area. In other words, breast cancer that spread to the liver became liver cancer. This is in error and is not the case. The cancer did not become liver cancer because it spread to this area of the body. It is still breast cancer, but has metastasized (spread) to the liver. The cancer does keep its name based upon its point of origin and its retention of tumor makeup at its initial site. In other words, the tumor on the liver is a breast cancer tumor. It is not a new incident of cancer when this happens.

Otherwise, if it was liver cancer, it would be a new incident of cancer and would not be categorized as having spread (metastasized) there.

Distant mets is when the cancer has spread to a distant part in the body beyond the nearby lymph nodes. Spread to the lung or liver would fall into the category of distant metastasis, based on its distance from the breast.

Can a person have two types of cancer at once in different places? Yes, they could. However, when we talk about metastasis, it does rule out that they are same, because they are different; separate incidents, in that case and do not fit into the category of having spread there.

Coping with recurrent and or metastatic breast cancer (advanced disease) is difficult, but not hopeless. There is a great deal of resources available to those living with metastatic breast cancer for support, advocacy and clinical trials (see additional resources page).

Author's Notes

In closing, because this book is a first of many to come and dedicated to my mother. I would be remiss not to pay her tribute here and now. She is currently battling two forms of stomach cancer. Although, her spirit remains high, she was diagnosed approximately three years ago and given a poor prognosis at pre-op. However, post-op she is amazing her doctors and continues to live independently and better than expected. This is where faith comes in and God is truly good.

My mother has weathered a number of the storms of life and had many victories and successes, despite her humble beginnings. She is the eldest of our family still living. She had her first bout with cancer over thirty years ago, when she was diagnosed with breast cancer. When I was diagnosed, I had nearly forgotten she too has a history of breast cancer. Back then my mother didn't talk about her cancer experience at all. This time was different I was blessed with being able to assist my mother through surgery and her transition home from the hospital. Although stubborn at times her will is commendable and resilient. Her life and stamina is a testimony of what God can and will do when we trust him.

As I was writing this I was reminded of what my friend Cynthia said when I mentioned God in this manner shortly after my diagnosis. My guess was that, because I had cancer I should not be speaking on His goodness due to my situation. In the middle of my sentence, she abruptly interrupted with some gibberish about it. She said "Girl..." I, with eyebrows raised exclaimed, "what!?" and she answered "if I were you I would not be talking about how good God is." After she finished I shared with her that "I know God can prevent events, even if He doesn't cause them", "He can intervene should He choose to." But my take on it was that because He didn't, He was obviously going to do something else with it and He has. I had already moved passed disappointment by then and this was not the time for any foolishness. God can do anything but fail.

"It almost seems Impossible until it is done."

(Nelson Mandela)

BREAST CANCER RESOURCES AND MORE INFORMATION

AMERICAN CANCER SOCIETY	(800) 227-2345
BECKSTRAND	(949) 955-0099
BREAST CANCER ANGELS	(714) 898-8900
CANCER CARE	(800) 813-4673
CANCER LEGAL RESOURCES	(866) 999-3752
CENTER FOR DISEASE CONTROL	(800) 232-4636
FERTILE HOPE	(855) 220-7777
LIVING BEYOND BREAST CANCER	(855) 807-6386
PROJECT ANGEL FOOD	(323) 845-1800
MY SISTER MY FRIEND BREAST CANCER SUPPORT	(866) 542-6312
NATIONAL CANCER INSTITUTE	(800) 422-6237
SIMMS/MANN – UCLA CENTER FOR INTEGRATIVE ONCOLOGY	(310) 794-6644
SISTERS BREAST CANCER SURVIVORS NETWORK	(323) 759-0200
SISTERS NETWORK NATIONAL	(866) 781-1808
THE G.R.E.E.N. FOUNDATION	(714) 507-0338
WOMEN OF ESSENCE	(310) 537-8227
YOUNG SURVIVORS COALITION	(877) 973-1011
Y-ME	(530) 753-3940

METASTATIC BREAST CANCER NETWORK (MBCN)
http://mbcn.org

ADVANCED BREAST CANCER COMMUNITY
http://www.advancedbreastcancercommunity.org/tools-and-support/

ADVANCEDBC.ORG – METASTATIC BREAST CANCER INFORMATION
AND SUPPORT FOR PATIENTS, FAMILY
... publications and online and telephone support groups without cost.

THE META CANCER FOUNDATION
http://metacancer.org

METAVIVOR - METASTATIC BREAST CANCER AWARENESS AND
RESEARCH   *http://www.metavivor.org*

METASTATIC BREAST CANCER - LIVING BEYOND BREAST CANCER
http://www.lbbc.org/Audiences/Metastatic-Breast-Cancer

METASTATIC BREAST CANCER PATIENT SUPPORT GROUP @
CANCER CARE *http://www.cancercare.org/support_groups/44-metastatic_
breast_cancer_patient_support_group*

BREASTCANCER.ORG
http://www.breastcancer.org/symptoms/types/recur_metast

ADVANCEDBC.ORG
http://www.bcrecovery.org/pages/Metastatic-Breast-Cancer-Resources.php

LIVING WITH ADVANCED OR METASTATIC BREAST CANCER
http://www.oncolink.org/types/article.cfm?c=68&id=9678

REFERENCES

Price, B. R. (1997). *Through the Fire, Through the Water: My Triumph Over Cancer.* Los Angeles: Faith One Publishers.

Lewis, C. S. (2009). *The Problem of Pain.* Pymble, NSW: Harper Collins e-books.

Alcorn, R. C. (2010). *If God is Good Why Do We Hurt?* Colorado Springs, Colo.: Multnomah Books.

Support Groups. nd. *In Wikipedia.* Retrieved May 15, 2014 from http://en.wikipedia.org/wiki/Support Groups.

American College of Radiology - *Radiology Society of North America. Patient Safety: Radiation Exposure in X-ray and CT Examinations.* Accessed at ww.radiologyinfo.org/en/safety/index.cfm?pg=sfty_xray on December 2, 2013.

Health Wheel, Creative Commons 2.0, http://*www.alreadypretty.com/wp-content/uploads/2012health_wheel.jpg. Already Pretty is licensed under a Creative Commons Attribution.*

END NOTES

[ii] American Cancer Society - Mammograms and Other Breast Imaging Tests
http://www.cancer.org/treatment/understandingyourdiagnosis/examsandtestdescriptions/mammogramsandotherbreastimagingprocedures/mammograms-and-other-breast-imaging-procedures-newer-br-imaging-tests

[iii] WebMD – *"Breast Cancer Signs and Symptoms"*
   Source: The American Cancer Society

[v] American Cancer Society - *Living With Uncertainty: The Fear of Cancer Recurrence* - Cancer.org

[vi] FDA-*Protecting America's Health Through Human Drugs*
A Special Report From the *FDA Consumer Magazine* and the
FDA Center for Drug Evaluation and Research Fourth Edition
/ January 2006.

[vii] Socioeconomic Status. (n.d.) *The American Heritage® New Dictionary of Cultural Literacy, Third Edition.* Retrieved June 23, 2014, from Dictionary.com website: h*ttp://dictionary.reference.com/browse/socioeconomic status*

[viii] *Socioeconomic Status (SES) - Adapted from APA's Socioeconomic Status American Psychological Association, Task Force on Socioeconomic Status. (2007).* Report of the APA Task Force on Socioeconomic Status. Washington, DC: American Psychological Association.

[ix] About.Com – Health
(http://firstaid.about.com/od/bleedingcontrol/f/11_How-Long-Does-a-Tetanus-Shot-Last.htm)

[x] Medline Plus – *Trusted Health Information For You*
Source: National Cancer Institute. *Nutrition in cancer care (PDQ).* November 13, 2011. Accessed May 19, 2012.
h*ttp://www.nlm.nih.gov/medlineplus/ency/patientinstructions/000061.htm)*

[xx] *Lymphatic System: Facts, Functions & Diseases*
Kim Ann Zimmermann, Live Science Contributor | February 08, 2013, 3:22 pm ET

ABOUT THE AUTHOR

Antoinette Greer has over twelve years of survivorship and is a Co-Founder of My Sister My Friend Breast Cancer Support. The Los Angeles native was a resident of Long Beach, California when diagnosed with breast cancer in 2002. At the age of forty, she underwent a Modified Radical Mastectomy, six months of chemotherapy and twenty-six treatments of radiation. It was during this time that she learned the women in her community faced marginal challenges in areas such as access to care, cultural competence and overall survival of the disease. One year post treatment, she gathered together with three other survivors and formed an Affiliate Chapter of Sisters Network, an African American Breast Cancer Survivorship Organization, recognized nationally for helping women in their communities. The group later became My Sister My Friend Breast Cancer Support in 2006. Antoinette sought to take charge of the needs of women treating in her community through program development, that these women might not slip through the cracks and re-enter the mainstream.

She is a volunteer, patient advocate and spokesperson for the American Cancer Society and a strong collaborator for navigational screening services. She is a former Counselor for the Spirit Project with M.D. Anderson Cancer Center and a volunteer to St Mary Medical Center's Community Benefits-Community Outreach Staff. She is a recipient of the Phenomenal Woman Award presented by the NAACP's Long Beach Affiliate, the John Lea Community Service Award, the Patient in Courage Award, presented by the American Cancer Society, the Partners in Education Award from the CUSD and several other superior performance awards regarding the spirit of excellence in her work. The group acts as a current Co-Sponsor of the Annual Body & Soul; A Wellness Forum and supports women referred to the group by clinics and hospitals throughout Los Angeles County. Antoinette continues to develop educational outreach and support programs that foster meeting the individual, basic needs of women battling the disease and in support of early detection.

ORDER BOOKS

To contact Antoinette Greer or to order books:
ASK ANTOINETTE
C/O
Antoinette Greer
P.O. BOX 61135
LOS ANGELES, CA 90061

ONLINE SALES VISIT
WWW.ASKANTOINETTE.COM
OR AMAZON.COM

OTHER BOOKS FORTHCOMING BY THIS AUTHOR:

BETWEEN SISTERS

TEN DAYS FOR CULTIVATING CHANGE: A SPIRITUAL
JOURNEY JOURNAL FOR BREAST CANCER SURVIVORS

WHO REALLY CARES: FACING FUNDING AND ACCESS TO
CARE ISSUES FOR MINORITIES AND VULNERABLE
POPULATIONS

www.ingramcontent.com/pod-product-compliance
Lightning Source LLC
Chambersburg PA
CBHW060219290526
45789CB00003B/1331